Chair Yoga

Learn Simple Exercises on Chair, Reduce Stress from Your Body and Improve Health While Sitting

John McCall

Table of Contents

Introduction

Chair yoga is part of the hatha branch of yoga. Hatha relates to yoga of the body, including poses, breathing, and meditation. Yoga techniques help you create a better harmony between your body, mind, and spirit. They also provide you with a low-impact way to increase strength, flexibility, and balance, while teaching you how relax.

Chair yoga can be practiced by adults of any age or physical condition. As you will see throughout this book, certain poses are not recommended for individuals with specific physical conditions. Other poses can be practiced with modifications. Listen to your body; if your body is uncomfortable with a certain pose, back off and find out why.

Your mind, emotions, and body are tightly intertwined. What affects one will impact the other. It is not uncommon for someone to consult a doctor when his or her emotions refuse to respond to professional counseling. In the same way, if physical conditions don't respond to yoga, a trip to the doctor may be a good idea.

Sometimes a visit with a trained yoga instructor can correct positioning that would otherwise cause harm, or would prevent you from experiencing the full benefits of a specific pose. However, little potential harm can come from practicing the beginner-level poses in this book, if you follow the instructions and honor the restrictions that are given for each one. Feel free to let these pages be your introduction to the wonderful and challenging world of yoga.

Women and Children

Some experts recommend that women who are nursing, pregnant, or menstruating should forego yoga entirely, but most admit that while the most strenuous poses, especially inversions, should be avoided during menstruation and pregnancy, some of the gentler asanas can actually be beneficial. In this book you will discover poses that are frequently used to relieve menstrual pain, address the symptoms of menopause, and support a woman's body during pregnancy.

Nursing mothers often benefit from poses that can support the muscles used to hold a baby while nursing, avoiding backache and injury caused by the repetitive motions of lifting and carrying a baby. It can also relieve postpartum depression and help both mother and baby relax during those first few weeks of adjusting to breastfeeding. Some mothers even opt to nurse their infants while they perform various yoga poses.

Chapter 2: Benefits of Health and Fitness

Exercise promotes the human body in many different ways such as shielding you from heart disease, stroke, and even high blood pressure. You can even alleviate your back pain, circulation issues, and prevent obesity. For those who have packed on a few pounds, physical exercise should be done daily to see results that can be a great benefit to your health. Health and fitness experts have recommended that you should engage in twenty to thirty minutes of exercise, mainly aerobic activity. Three times each week is sufficient for this and if you want greater results, stack up some more days.

For those who haven't been active for quite a while, they'll want to work their way up by practicing an activity that is not very strenuous. A brisk walk or some light swimming is suggested for those who want to start off at a slow pace and build their fitness schedule from there. This can easily lead up to other activities like running, soccer, or even volleyball.

With health and fitness, you can condition your body and prepare for the future. It's been proven that those who exercise and eat right have increased their chances of living longer, compared to those who don't.

The risk of dying prematurely is reduced.

Your risk of heart disease has been greatly reduced.

You won't be likely to develop diabetes.

High blood pressure is decreased for those who exercise.

Great for weight management.

Help develop and even maintain your muscles and joints.

Circulates the blood in the body, causing fewer clots.

Reduces your stress by promoting healthy psychological well-being.

Chapter 3: The Specific Benefits of Exercise

Heart Disease / Stroke: Did you know that keeping up with your daily physical activity can decrease your chances of heart disease or stroke? The reason why is because by exercising, you are strengthening the muscle of your heart. This also allows you to lower your blood pressure and raise something called HDL. This is just an acronym for high-density lipoprotein or otherwise known as "great cholesterol." It will improve your blood flow and even increase the capacity of your heart.

High blood pressure: Doing daily physical activity can contribute to reducing blood pressure in most individuals. Also, it will reduce your body fat which is heavily linked to high blood pressure.

Diabetes: When reducing your body fat, exercise can prevent and maintain any diabetes that you've acquired.

Obesity: Constant, daily physical activity has been known to reduce body fat. Every time you run or make any movement, you are burning calories. When you add this to proper nutrition, your body fat will begin to disappear. People who have obesity have a harder time moving and doing things, even around the house.

Back Pain: When you increase your muscle strength and build up endurance with working out, running, or aerobics - it can help with your posture. Also, it will allow you to be more flexible which means your back pain won't be as bad as it was before.

Precautions

As much as chair yoga is a gentle, safe road to take toward fitness, please follow the advice of your physician on exercises that you should or should not do.

Yoga emphasizes "listening to the body." The exercises and poses are sometimes challenging, but should never be practiced to the point of pain. There are many ways to achieve the same stretch or the same objective in yoga, so always feel free to skip a pose and move on to the next one. Before doing any endurance exercises or deep stretches, please warm up.

Pay special attention to the following conditions:

Disc issues or spinal degeneration – When bending forward from the waist, go only about 45 degrees (not chest to thighs).

Spinal arthritis/bone spurs and degeneration – When bending backward, keep the head straight rather than allowing the head to fall back.

High or low blood pressure – On postures that move the head and/or chest up or down, move slowly to allow for the body to adjust to the change.

The above is a list of the most common contraindications. Most importantly, listen to your body and your physician.

Principles of Yoga

Although the following five principles encompass ideas from all styles of yoga, they originate from Sivananda, as taught by Swami Vishnu-devananda in *The Complete Illustrated Book of Yoga*:

1. PROPER EXERCISE: Yoga exercises are performed slowly, gently, and with awareness. Keep in mind that all bodies are different.

2. PROPER BREATHING: Deep breathing helps to nourish and strengthen the body.

3. PROPER RELAXATION: Releasing tension through relaxation is essential for a healthy body. Many yoga students consider complete relaxation of the body and mind to be most difficult, but important to work toward.

4. PROPER DIET: Simple, nutritious foods are basic for good health. A true yoga diet is a vegetarian diet.

5. POSITIVE THINKING and MEDITATION: Positive thinking leads to contentment—being thankful for who you are, what you can do, and what you have. There is no need to envy what others can do or what others have. Make peace with the past and move forward.

Chapter 4: Breathing exercises

Correct breathing is one of yoga's key principles. The outcome of relaxation can quickly be obtained through basic breathing exercises. It also helps you maintain focus, heat in the body, and good circulation throughout your practice. These exercises are also beneficial for the respiratory, circulatory, and nervous systems.

Yoga breathing is usually done through the nostrils, which helps keep heat in the body as opposed to most aerobic exercise where you usually exhale through the mouth to help cool the body.

Keep in mind that when one is becoming accustomed to breathing techniques, it is common to become a bit light-headed, dizzy, or tense. Try these techniques a little at a time and with a relaxed and open mind. If you experience anything uncomfortable, then stop and try again another time.

ABDOMINAL BREATHING

Inhale deeply through your nose. Allow the abdomen to expand, which helps lower your diaphragm, and bring oxygen into the base of the lungs. Exhale through your nose. Contract your abdominal muscles, pull your abdomen in, and raise the diaphragm, pushing out air.

If this is new to you it will feel awkward at first. Try the exercise while lying on your back with one hand over your belly button. Feel the rise and fall of your abdomen.

COMPLETE BREATH

Beginning with the abdominal breath, focus on this outward and inward movement of the belly for a few breaths. When this feels comfortable, focus on bringing this expansion upward toward the chest on the inhale as if you were filling up a pitcher with water. On the exhalations, the water is draining out of the pitcher.

ALTERNATE NOSTRIL BREATHING I

You can experiment with many variations of Alternate Nostril Breathing. Here is one of the simpler versions: Hold up your right hand. Fold down your index and middle fingers. You will use your thumb and fingers to gently seal your nostrils closed. Close off your right nostril with your thumb while you inhale through your left nostril. Close off your left nostril with your fingers. Release the right nostril and exhale through your right nostril. Inhale through the right nostril. Close right, release left, and then exhale through the left nostril. Continue back and forth for a minute or longer. Your breathing should be relaxed and rhythmic.

ALTERNATE NOSTRIL BREATHING II

Hold up your right hand. Fold down your index and middle fingers. (You will be using your thumb and ring finger to hold down nostrils.) If you find this too uncomfortable, just use your thumb and index fingers. Close off your left nostril with your fingers. Inhale through your right nostril for a count of four. Lift your fingers and close your right nostril with your thumb. Exhale to a count of eight. Try this for about a minute and then switch sides. Close off your right nostril with your thumb, inhaling through your left nostril for a count of four. Lift your thumb and close off your left nostril with your fingers. Exhale to a count of eight.

ALTERNATE NOSTRIL BREATHING III

This exercise helps to clear and calm the mind. [Note: Pregnant woman should check with their doctor before retaining the breath.] Close off your right nostril with your thumb, and inhale to a count of four. Close off your left nostril with your fingers, holding your breath for a count of sixteen. Lift your thumb, and exhale for a count of eight. Inhale to a count of four. Close and hold for a count of sixteen. With fingers up, exhale for a count of eight. Continue for four or more rounds, and then sit for a few moments, relaxing your body and mind.

Chapter 5: How to Begin

It may be helpful to skim through the entire book first before trying to physically do each pose. Getting familiar with the poses first will make your practice smoother and more enjoyable.

Select a sturdy, armless, straight-back chair that allows you to put your feet flat on the floor. Wear comfortable clothing. You may choose to remove your shoes and socks. A quiet area, free from distractions, is ideal. Relaxing music may enhance your practice.

SITTING POSTURES

There are two ways to sit in your chair throughout your yoga practice. The first, Relaxing Posture, is meant for resting the body. The other is a Yogic Posture, from which you start a pose.

RELAXING POSTURE

Sit all the way back in your chair with your feet resting comfortably on the floor. Let your hands rest on your thighs, either palms up or down. Close your eyes or just allow your gaze to drop softly ahead of you.

Use relaxing posture to rest during your practice or in between poses. Relaxing between postures helps you prepare for moving again.

YOGIC POSTURE

Begin each posture by sitting tall with your back away from the back of the chair. Lengthen through the spine with your chest out and abs in. Imagine that you are being lifted from the very top of your head up to the ceiling. Think of this as your working posture.

DRISHTI

Many yoga students wonder where they are supposed to look when they are in a pose. Yogis call the focus of the eyes during a pose or meditation a *drishti*. The famous yogi and founder of Ashtanga Yoga, Sri K. Pattabhi Jois, popularized drishti techniques. Think of your drishti as where you should gaze during a pose. In this book, we often suggest that you look upward, straight out over your fingertips or wherever the neck and head is comfortable, depending on the pose. You may also practice many poses with your eyes closed or softly focusing on the floor.

BREATHING AND RELAXING

Using your breath when working in the postures adds to the experience. Keep in mind that relaxed muscles stretch. As you linger in a pose, try relaxing your body. With your exhale, sink deeper into the posture. Typically, you exhale to lower into a pose and inhale to rise out of, or release, a pose. Approach challenging poses with patience and care.

INTENTION

You can set an intention before you start each yoga session. This might be what you wish to accomplish, change, or feel as a result of your practice. It could also be a physical attribute, such as "I am going to feel more flexible after class today," or a mental or emotional intention, such as "I am going to stop worrying about things over which I have no control" or "I am going to have a softer heart with those I love." You might decide to dedicate your workout to someone who is on your mind.

Next, try to clear your mind of all busy thoughts. Leave the past behind, and try not to think ahead to the future. Focus on the present moment.

Chapter 6: Warm Up Postures

The warm-up is intended to move each joint through a comfortable range of motion and increase the blood flow in your muscles, preparing them for longer-held and more challenging postures.

LOWER BODY
KNEE LIFTS

Sit tall with your hands at your side. Inhale and lift your right knee up. Exhale and lower your leg. Repeat four times and then switch to your left leg.

KNEE CROSS AND ROTATE

Inhale and lift your right knee up. Exhale and cross your right knee over your left leg. Inhale and lift your right knee back up. Exhale and uncross the knee, putting your foot down. Repeat four times and then switch to your left leg.

Inhale and lift your right knee up. Exhale, rotating your lifted knee to your right side. Inhale, moving your knee back to center and exhale your leg down. Repeat four times and then switch to your left leg.

KNEE TO CHEST

Inhale your right knee to your chest and place your foot in the chair or hold your shin with your hands. Exhale. Inhale your chin to the ceiling. Exhale your chin to your chest. Breathe into your lower back, and then breathe into your middle back. Inhale into your shoulder blades, and exhale down your arms. Inhale your chin to the ceiling. Exhale as you lower your leg and relax your body. Repeat with your left leg.

LEG EXTENSIONS

Inhale and lift one knee high, and then straighten your leg. Exhale and bend your knee, and then lower your foot to the floor. Repeat three to six times on each leg.

ANKLE ROTATIONS

Inhale both feet up until your legs are straight. Rotate your feet several times, and then reverse the rotation. Point and flex your feet several times. With your feet flexed, touch your toes together as your heels splay out, and then touch your heels together as your toes splay out. Repeat several times. End with several flutter kicks.

TOE AND HEEL TAPPING

With feet flat on the floor, challenge the left and right sides of the brain by tapping the heel of your left foot at the same time that you tap the toes of your right foot. Switch to right heel and left toes.

FOOT ROTATIONS

Start with feet flat on the floor, and then rise up on your toes. Roll around to the outside of your feet, back to your heels, and to the inside of your feet. Repeat several times, and then reverse directions.

FOOT PRESSES

With feet hip width apart, point toes toward the sky. Hold for a few seconds, then bring the toes down and lift both heels. Hold for a few seconds.

20. SUN SALUTATION

Use this sequence as a way to warm up. Take your knees apart slightly wider than hip width. Inhaling, sweep your arms out to your sides and overhead. Exhaling, place your hands on your thighs as you lean forward, flattening your back. Inhale and then exhale as you fold over, letting your hands rest on your shins or the floor. Inhale and come back up with a flat back, bringing your hands back to your thighs. Exhale as you sit back in your chair and relax.

UPPER BODY
SHOULDER SHRUGS

Inhale as you lift your shoulders up high toward your ears. Exhale and drop your shoulders as low as you can.

SHOULDER ROLLS
Breathe comfortably as you roll your shoulders in three circles forward and then in three circles backward.

SHOULDER RELEASE

Inhale and place your fingertips on your shoulders. Exhale and touch your elbows together in front of your body. Inhale and pull your elbows back as far as you can comfortably.

SIDE-TO-SIDE NECK WARM-UP

Inhale and turn your head to the right (as if trying to look over your shoulder). Exhale and turn your head back to center. Inhale and turn your head to the left. Exhale and turn your head back to center.

TURTLE NECK

Sitting tall, move your head straight forward, keeping your chin parallel to the floor. Then move your head back, centering it over the spine.

NECK PENDULUM

Inhale and sit up as tall as you can. Exhaling, gently drop your chin to your chest. Inhaling, roll your right ear to your right shoulder. Exhaling, drop your chin to your chest. Inhaling, roll your left ear to your left shoulder. Exhaling, drop your chin to your chest. Inhale and come back to center.

HALF MOON

Bring your arms overhead with your palms together. Inhale, stretch, and reach up as tall as you can. Exhale as you bend gently to the right. Inhale, stretch, and reach up tall. Exhale as you bend gently to the left. Inhale as you stretch tall again.

TORSO

CAT/COW

Rest your hands on your thighs. Exhale as you look to your navel, rounding your back and dropping your chin to your chest. Inhale and lengthen your spine, bending back slightly and pressing your chest and belly forward.

FLOWING AIRPLANE

Inhaling, reach your arms overhead. Exhale as you bring your chest forward toward your thighs, stretching your arms back behind you, parallel to the floor.

FLOWING SPINAL TWIST

Starting with your hands at your sides, inhale as you raise your arms overhead. Exhale as you turn to the right. Drop your left hand outside your right knee and hold the back of the chair by the seat with your right hand. Inhale as you raise your arms overhead and repeat on the left side.

CIRCLING ARMS

Place your hands together at your heart center. Circle your arms out to your sides and overhead, bringing palms back together. Exhale as you lower your arms down to your heart center. After repeating three times, reverse directions.

Starting at your heart center, inhale as you raise your arms overhead, and then exhale as you circle down, bringing your hands to your heart center again. Repeat three times.

Chapter 7: Endurance and Strength Postures

For all the postures below, sit toward the front of your chair. Take three to five breaths per exercise. Most importantly, do not hold your breath while doing any postures.

Standing Postures

MOUNTAIN POSE (the foundation of all standing poses)

Like many other poses, those that appear to be "easy" or "simple" often provide great opportunity for deep, focused physical and mental work. Try the simple version of Mountain below and then use some of the bulleted tips for future practices. Stand tall with your feet about hip distance apart and your arms at your sides, slightly away from your body. Keep your chest high, abs in, and shoulders back and relaxed. Lift and spread your toes and the balls of your feet, and then lay them softly down on the floor. Rock back and forth and from side to side. Gradually reduce this swaying to a standstill, with your weight balanced evenly on your feet.

- Put a tiny bend in your knees and see if you feel your back and abdominal muscles work even harder.
- Lengthen your spine, reaching the crown of your head toward the sky while keeping your shoulders back and down.
- Imagine three points on the bottom of each foot—one on the heel and the other two on each side of the ball of the foot. Root these six points down, keeping the natural arches in your feet.
- Slightly or completely close your eyes to challenge your balance. Build confidence in this

balance as you think about what it feels like to be a mountain.
- Visualize electrically charged roots moving down from the bottom of the feet and fingertips into the Earth and from the crown of the head upward.

Variation: Walk around your chair several times while engaging the principles of Mountain Pose. A little walk in Mountain Pose may help you be more aware of your walking posture.

CAT/COW
Bend your knees, getting into a semi-squat position. Place your hands on your thighs just above your knees. Exhale as you look to your navel and round your back like a scared cat. Inhale as you look up, pressing your tailbone out and your chest forward, swaying your back. Repeat several times in a flowing manner.

ARM CIRCLES
With arms out in a T-shape and palms facing the floor, slowly make small circles in a forward motion. Try to keep the shoulders down and relaxed as you start making the circles bigger. Without lowering the arms, switch directions, starting with small circles. After several breaths, make the circles bigger. Shake your arms gently after you bring them down to your sides.

PRAYER SQUAT FLOW
Plant feet firmly onto floor with legs wide apart and toes pointed slightly outward. Inhaling, raise your arms out to the sides and then overhead. Exhaling, bend your knees into a wide-legged squat and lean forward, letting your

arms sweep down and out to your sides, then to the space between your knees, with hands crossing. Inhaling, sweep your arms out and up in a circling motion overhead as you straighten your legs. Continue this flow for as many rounds as you like.

Variation: Keep your torso more upright throughout the flow. To challenge your balance, try closing your eyes for a few rounds.

HALF MOON

Bring your arms overhead with your palms together. Inhale as you stretch up as tall as you can. Exhaling, bend gently to the right. Inhaling, return to center. Exhaling, bend gently to the left. Inhaling, return to center. Repeat two or three times, and then rest your arms at your sides.

TRIANGLE

Starting from Mountain Pose, separate your feet at least two feet apart, making them parallel. Inhale your left arm up beside your left ear. Exhale and bend to your right side, allowing your right hand to slide down your leg. Avoid bending forward, and keep your hips squared. Hold for three or more breaths. Return to center, and then switch to your right. Repeat at least twice.

Variation: With feet at least two feet apart, point your left foot to the left, and rotate your right heel slightly to the right. Inhale as you lift your arms up in a T-position. Exhale as you lower your right hand down your right leg, either above or below your knee, and your left hand up to the sky. Keep your left shoulder back, and avoid bending forward. Try to keep both sides of your body lengthened. Repeat on the right side.

REVOLVED TRIANGLE

Starting from Mountain Pose, separate your feet wider than shoulder width apart, with both feet facing forward. Raise your arms to shoulder height in a T-position. Turn to the right, bend from the hip, and exhale down, bringing your left hand to your right leg, as low as possible, with both legs straight. Hold for three or more breaths. Inhale up. Turn to the left and repeat.

WARRIOR I

Stand behind your chair. Take your feet into a stance at least two feet apart. Point your right foot to the right, and rotate your left heel slightly to the left. Turn your torso to the right, and bend your right knee slightly. Inhale and bring both arms straight up (or just the right arm if you are holding onto the chair back), aiming your fingers and gaze to where the ceiling and wall meet, or higher. Hold for a few breaths.

WARRIOR II

Starting from Warrior I, turn your torso to the front, bringing one or both arms down to shoulder height, with the palms down. Look just over your right fingertips. Try to relax your shoulders and square them to the front. Hold for a few breaths.

REVERSED WARRIOR

Starting from Warrior II, allow your left hand to rest on your left hip or leg. Rotate your right palm up, and then reach your right hand toward the ceiling. Keep your gaze upward toward your hand. Hold for a few breaths.

SIDE-ANGLE WARRIOR

Starting from Reverse Warrior, lean over and rest your right arm on your right thigh. Inhale your left arm straight overhead. Look toward your left hand. Hold for a few breaths.

Turn back to center. Repeat all of the Warrior postures on your left side.

CAMEL

Stand with feet about hip width apart. Place your palms against your lower back on each side of your spine. Expand your chest, lifting your chin slightly. Press elbows toward one another. Hold for a few breaths and then release.

DOWNDOG

Downdog is a staple pose for many yoga classes. Starting behind your chair, grasp the chair back. Step back until your hips are stacked over your feet. Think of yourself as if you are an upside-down L or 90-degree angle. Your arms should be straight out from your shoulders. Enjoy stretching through your shoulders and the backs of your legs. Try to flatten the back as much as possible, and bring your head between your upper arms.

LEG RAISE

Stand behind your chair. Place one hand on the chair back for balance, if necessary. Slowly inhale your right leg to the side. Hold for two to three breaths, and then slowly exhale your leg down. Repeat the exercise about four times for each leg. Now try the exercise with your leg extending behind you (four times for each leg). Then step to the side of your chair, extending your leg to the front (again, four times for each leg). Remember to keep your leg straight and the knee soft.

FORWARD BEND

In one variation, you stretch more through your back and spine, and in the other, you stretch more through your hamstrings.

For the back and spine:

Stand up tall with your feet together. Inhale your arms straight up to the ceiling. Exhale and slowly bend forward from your hips, letting your arms move out to your sides as you move toward the floor. Bend your knees so your hands can reach the floor. Allow your torso to rest on your thighs. Let your spine elongate and stretch.

For the hamstrings:

Stand up tall with your feet together. Inhale your arms straight up to the ceiling. Exhale and slowly bend forward from your hips. Sweep your arms across the ceiling and down the wall. Keep your legs straight, but avoid locking your knees. Allow your arms to fall loose, with the top of your head facing the floor. Breathe naturally, allowing your body to lower a little more with each exhale. Slowly roll up to a standing posture.

Balance Postures

Practice balance because it is your best defense against a fall. Keep in mind that you do simple balance every time you take a step. You only need the chair to get into some balancing postures. Hold the chair to begin, and then let go once you are in the pose. If you feel unsteady when balancing on one leg, put your other foot down. Reaching for a chair is not advised. It is unlikely that a chair will be handy when you need one, but your foot is always with you. In our teaching experience, we found that when you make a habit of putting your foot down instead of depending on a chair, you are much safer from a fall.

For balance postures, it helps to relax the body and focus your eyes on something that does not move.

BALANCE ON TOES

Rise up gently on your toes. Bring hands to your heart center and then overhead, with your palms together. Hold for three or four breaths.

FLAMINGO

Alternate picking up your right and left foot several times. Increase the length of time you hold your balance.

KNEE LIFTS

Bring your right knee up in front, straighten your leg, bend again, and put it down. Repeat with your left knee.

KNEE TO CHEST

Bring your right knee up in front, hold onto your shin, and gently pull your knee into your chest. Hold for three or four breaths. Repeat with your left knee.

KNEE UP TWIST

Stand beside your chair. Inhale your left knee up, and extend your arms out in a T-shape. Turn to the left, bringing your left hand to the back and your right hand to the front. Hold for a few breaths. Try looking toward your left hand. Repeat on the other side.

TREE

Standing tall, extend your right leg to the side, with your toe touching the floor. Slide your heel to your left ankle. Raise your foot up to the calf or thigh, keeping the knee pressed to the side.

Avoid putting the foot by the knee. You might have your arms in T-position, hands at your heart center, or overhead. Hold the posture for a few breaths, and then repeat on the left.

DANCER'S POSE

Stand tall. Hold the back of the chair with your left hand. If needed, bend your right knee and grasp your right ankle with your right hand. When you feel in balance, inhale the left hand to the ceiling. Repeat on the other side.

DANCER WITH HALF BOW

Starting from Dancer's Pose, gently push your foot away from your body into a bow, then start leaning forward until your knee and head are close to level with the chair back. Repeat on the other side.

WARRIOR III

Standing beside your chair, hold the chair back with your right hand, if needed. Keep the chair at arm's length. Stretch your left hand out making a half T-shape. Lean forward as you raise your right leg until your body is parallel to the floor. When you feel confident, bring your left hand out to complete the T and balance. Repeat on the other side.

CHAIR SQUAT

Reach your arms straight out in front of you, bend your knees, and lower your hips as if you are sitting down onto a chair. Hold the posture for a few breaths. Now rise up on your toes and hold for a few breaths.

CHAIR SQUAT ON ONE LEG

Place your right ankle just above your left knee. Reach your arms straight out in front of you or bring your hands to heart center in prayer position while bending your knees and lowering your hips as if you are sitting down onto a chair. Hold this posture for a few breaths. Repeat on your other leg.

Eye Witness

Eye exercises strengthen the extraocular muscles of the eyes and reduce tension. Keep your head and torso still while doing these exercises.

UP-DOWN RIGHT-LEFT

Look up and look down three times, close your eyes, and breathe. Look to the right and look to the left three times, close your eyes, and breathe.

DIAGONAL RIGHT-LEFT

Look up diagonally to the right and diagonally down to the left three times, close your eyes, and breathe. Look up diagonally to the left and diagonally down to the right three times, close your eyes, and breathe.

AROUND THE CLOCK

Slowly look around the clock three times starting at twelve o'clock, then around to three, down to six, around to nine, and back up to twelve. Close your eyes and breathe. Slowly look around the clock counter clockwise three times starting at twelve o'clock, then around to nine, down to six, around to three, and then back up to twelve. Close your eyes and breathe.

FINGER GAZE

Starting with your index finger on the tip of your nose, slowly extend your arm and then return it to the start position, continually following your finger with your eyes. Lower your arm. Repeat three times. Close your eyes and breathe.

COVERED EYES

Remove glasses if needed. Rub the palms of your hands together, creating a little warmth. Close your eyes and place your hands on your cheekbones, covering but not touching your eyelids. Hold for three slow breaths. Lower your arms and relax the body.

Finger Exercises

Finger exercises are particularly good for arthritic finger joints.

FINGER FLEX

Stretch your fingers wide. Squeeze your fingertips down to the top pad of your hand, and then make a fist. Repeat twice.

FINGER SQUEEZE

Stretch your fingers wide. Beginning with your little fingers, bend each finger and push it into the top pad of your hand with your thumb.

FINGER STRETCHES

With your palm facing up, use other hand to gently pull each finger back one at a time toward the back of your hand; do not stretch thumb joint.

PULL AND TWIST

Starting with the little finger of your right hand, pull on your finger with your left hand, and then twist your finger away from you. Repeat on each of the other fingers.

JOINING

Place both hands down above your knees, with your thumb to the inside and your fingers to the outside. One at a time, bring each finger in to meet your thumb. Take each finger out again.

PARTING

Stretch your arms out in front of you, placing your palms together. Separate each finger, beginning with your little finger. Repeat twice.

THUMB TO FINGERS

Stretch the fingers out. Touch the base of your little fingers with your thumbs, and then slide your thumb out to the tip of your fingers. Repeat on each finger a few times.

Cool-Down Postures

The purpose of a cool-down is to return your body to its resting state.

BACK OF SHOULDER STRETCH

Bring your right arm across your chest. Place your left hand or arm above or below your right elbow. Gently hug your right arm close to your chest. Repeat on the other side.

MIDDLE OF BACK STRETCH

Bring your hands in front of your chest, interlacing fingers, so that you are looking at your palms. Reach your hands as far away as is comfortable, bringing your chin toward your chest. Gently round your back

ROCK THE BABY

Sit tall and place your right ankle on your left thigh. Flex the right foot and hold it with your left hand while holding your knee with the right hand. Swing your foot back and forth as if you are rocking a baby, and then draw the leg in toward your chest as if you are hugging the baby. Repeat with your other leg.

PIGEON

Sit tall and place your right ankle just above your left knee. Exhaling, bend forward from your hips, keeping your back flat. Hold for a few breaths. Inhaling, rise up into your Yogic Posture. Repeat on the other side.

If placing your ankle over your knee is difficult, sit forward in the chair, straighten your left leg and cross your right ankle over the left ankle, and then lean forward.

HAMSTRING STRETCH

Sit at the front edge of the chair and extend your right leg so it is almost straight (keep a slight bend in your knee). Your left foot should remain flat on the floor.

Gently lean forward from your hips until you feel a stretch in the back of your right thigh. For a calf stretch, stay in this position, but do not lean forward. Keep the right heel on the floor and pull your toes up toward your shins as much as possible.

INNER THIGH STRETCH
Sit to the front edge of the chair. Bring your feet and knees wide apart. Place hands on the inside of each thigh, gently pressing outward. Exhale forward, hinging from the hips and keeping a flat back. Lower as much as you like, and then inhale up. Repeat a few times.

WRIST RELEASE

Holding your arms in front of the body, circle hands at the wrists several times in each direction. Now point and flex the hands a few times and release.

FACIAL RELEASE

While relaxing the rest of your body, close your eyes and scrunch up the nose, forehead, lips, and eyes. Inhale as the tension builds. Exhale as you release and stretch your face back out, opening your mouth and moving your jaw gently back and forth.

LION POSE
With palms down over your knees, take a deep breath. As you exhale, open your eyes wide and stick your tongue far out of your mouth, expelling breath with a throaty whisper. Repeat two times.

71. SEATED FORWARD BEND
Sitting tall, inhale your arms overhead. Exhale as you bend forward until you are relaxing with your chest on your lap and

your arms dangling toward the floor. Remain here for a few breaths. Inhale as you slowly roll up one vertebra at a time: lower back, middle back, upper back, shoulder blades, shoulders, and head. Exhale to relax your body. Inhale and stretch out your arms and legs. Exhale and relax your body.

Seated Postures

CHAIR POSE

Hold the sides of the chair as you stand halfway out of your seat. Let the hips and thighs hover above the seat of the chair. Take hands to prayer position or extend them out straight in front of the body. Hold for a couple of breaths, and then sit carefully back onto your chair.

ARM CIRCLES

With arms out at your sides in a T-shape and palms facing the floor, slowly make small circles in a forward motion. Try to keep the shoulders down and relaxed. Start making the circles bigger. Without lowering the arms, switch directions, starting with small circles. After several breaths, make the circles bigger. Shake the arms gently after you bring them down to your sides.

TRIANGLE

Sit up tall. Inhale and lift your right arm straight up beside your ear and let your left arm hang down by your side or gently grasp the side of the chair. Looking straight ahead, exhale over to the left. Hold for three or more breaths. Return to center and then switch to your left arm. Repeat at least twice.

PRAYER SQUAT FLOW

Plant feet firmly onto the floor with legs wide apart and toes pointing slightly outward. Inhaling, raise your arms out to your sides, then overhead, crossing your arms. Exhaling, lean forward, letting your arms sweep down and out to the sides, then to the space between your knees, with hands briefly crossing. Inhaling, sweep arms out and up in a circling motion overhead. Continue to flow up and down for as many rounds as you like.

Variation: Keep your torso more upright throughout the flow.

ELBOW TO KNEE

Inhale and place your fingertips on your shoulders. Exhale and move your left elbow down to your right knee. Inhale up to your starting position. Exhale and move your right elbow to your left knee. Inhale and return to your starting position. Repeat several times.

Variation: Raise your knee as you exhale your elbow to your knee.

REVOLVED TRIANGLE

Sit tall with your feet wide apart. Place your right hand on your left knee as you lean slightly forward. Turn to the left and place your left hand on your hip. Hold for two or three breaths. Turn to the right and repeat.

Variation: For a deeper stretch, exhale as you slide your right hand down the left leg as low as possible.

Note: We describe the Warrior Poses in order from Warrior I, to Warrior II, to Reverse Warrior, and then to Side Angle. These poses flow nicely together. Once you become comfortable with the Warriors, try practicing them in various orders.

WARRIOR I

Spread your legs wide apart. Turn to your right, pushing your left leg back and pressing the ball of your foot onto the floor. Straighten your left leg as much as possible. Raise both arms up, aiming your fingers and gaze to where the ceiling meets the wall, or higher. Hold for a few breaths.

Variation: Turn your palms up.

WARRIOR II

Starting from Warrior I, turn your torso, allowing the hips and shoulders to face forward. Bring both arms down to shoulder height with your palms down. Let your toes point slightly to your right, and then press the outside edge of your left foot onto the floor. Look just past the fingertips on your right hand. Try to relax your shoulders and keep them square. Hold for a few breaths.

REVERSED WARRIOR

Starting from Warrior II, allow your left hand to rest on your left hip or your left leg while reaching your right hand toward the ceiling. Look toward your right hand. Hold for a few breaths.

SIDE-ANGLE WARRIOR

Starting from Reverse Warrior, lean to your right, resting your right arm on your right thigh. Inhale your left arm overhead. Gently press your left shoulder back. Look toward your left hand. Hold for a few breaths. Variation: Keep your left hand on your hip.

Turn back to center. Repeat all of the Warrior postures on your left side.

CAMEL

Place your palms against your lower back on each side of your
spine. Expand your chest, lifting your chin slightly. Press elbows
toward one another. Hold for a few breaths and then release.

GATE

Extend the left leg directly out to the side. Place your left hand
lightly on your left thigh. Inhale and lift your right arm up
toward the ceiling. Exhale and gently bend from the waist
toward the left. Repeat on the other side.

EAGLE

Cross your right leg over the left, trying to lock your right toes
behind your left leg. Spread the arms wide and then cross them
in front of the body to make an X by crossing the left arm on top
of the right so that your elbows are stacked one on top of the
other. Continue to wrap the forearms so that the palms and
fingers of each hand face one another, or so that the backs of
your hands touch. If this is not comfortable, just place your right
hand on your left shoulder and your left hand on your right
shoulder, giving yourself a hug. Repeat on the other side.

CHEST EXPANSION

Position feet hip width apart on the floor. Reach your arms
behind you to grasp the chair back. Inhale and gently bring your
chest forward until you feel a nice stretch in the front of your
shoulders and chest.

SPINAL TWIST

Let both legs turn to the right so that the left side of your body
faces the middle of the room. Place your right hand on the right
side of your seat back and the left on the left side. Gently look

toward your right shoulder. Allow your exhales to help you twist slightly deeper. Hold for five to seven breaths and then switch sides.

Foot and Toe Exercises

Your feet will thank you for giving them a little attention.

Begin with your right foot just above your left knee. After completing all of the following steps with the right foot, switch to the left foot.

PULL AND TWIST

Starting with your little toe, pull and twist each toe away from you.

MASSAGE

Pound on the sole of your foot with your left fist. Massage the ball of your foot with both thumbs.

CLASP

Place the palm of your left hand on the ball of your foot and lace your fingers through your toes.

Conclusion

The benefits of yoga are seemingly endless. You have seen how yoga can support your health by helping to improve your posture, by energizing your internal organs, by building strength and suppleness into your muscles, and by supporting your mental and spiritual well-being. Whatever your age, you can easily begin to practice yoga, using the instructions in this book. Even physical injuries and activity restrictions are no obstacle. With more than a hundred yoga forms from which to choose, many of which offer modifications to accommodate specific injuries, you will be able to stretch and strengthen your entire body. From beginning yoga positions to advanced poses, you now have access to the best of yoga, accessible practices that can bring increased health to every part of your body, mind, and spirit.

What we know today as yoga is a relatively recent form of the ancient practice. Introduced to America in the early 1900s, modern yoga is a mix of ancient Indian indigenous cultural practices and asanas, blended with modern gymnastics, physical therapy, and naturopathy.

Modern yoga was designed to help individuals become more self-aware, tuned into their body's needs, while opening up to both feelings and intuition. At the same time, it provides a full-body workout, including strength training and stretching. Contrary to popular belief, yoga is not a religion, although some people have included it as part of their religious practices. That is understandable, because this form of exercise is highly effective at removing distractions, calming the emotions, and clearing the mind, which lays a foundation for increased spiritual awareness. In this book, however, the focus will be on the physical aspects of yoga practice and how they can benefit your mind and your emotions.

The majority of yoga positions stimulate the glandular system, encouraging your internal organs to function efficiently. This exercise practice also promotes deep, controlled breathing, which encourages a centered, peaceful mind and a calm, alert spirit. The consistent practice of yoga can lead to many amazing physical, mental, and emotional benefits that you definitely don't want to miss out on!

Yoga comes in a variety of forms and levels of difficulty, ranging from very basic to extremely complex. Chair yoga focuses on posture, movement, and breathing. Other types of yoga focus intensely on breathing and meditation while others focus on aspects of wisdom and traditions associated with various forms of religion.

www.ingramcontent.com/pod-product-compliance
Lightning Source LLC
Chambersburg PA
CBHW070059260726
48658CB00002B/908